INTRODUCTION

When a man has issues with his sexual function, such as impotence or erectile dysfunction (ED), he may take tadalafil to help. Tadalafil is used to treat the symptoms of benign prostatic hyperplasia (BPH), which is an enlarged prostate, and when combined with sexual stimulation, it works by boosting blood flow to the penis, helping a man get and maintain an erection. Symptoms of benign prostatic hyperplasia (BPH) include incontinence, weak urine stream, and frequent or urgent urination (even in the middle of the night). It is believed that tadalafil relaxes the smooth muscles of the bladder and prostate. However, this medication does not provide protection against STDs such syphilis, gonorrhea, hepatitis B, or HIV. Engage in "safe sex" practices, such utilizing latex condoms. Further information should be sought from your physician or pharmacist.

THE CIALIS DOSAGE GUIDE

Before beginning treatment with tadalafil and at each refill, read the Patient Information Leaflet that may be available from your pharmacist. Consult your physician or pharmacist for clarification.

Follow your doctor's instructions regarding the proper way to take this medication by mouth. Never exceed a single daily dose of tadalafil.

This medicine should be swallowed whole, as directed by the manufacturer. But many of the same medications (immediate-release pills) are crushable. Take this medicine exactly as prescribed by your doctor. Your medical history, treatment efficacy, and any other drugs you are taking will determine the dosage. Never keep a secret from your doctor or pharmacist regarding the medications you use, whether they be prescription, over-the-counter, or herbal. Take this medication once daily or as prescribed by your doctor to alleviate the symptoms of benign prostatic hyperplasia. Consult your physician regarding the optimal duration of treatment for BPH symptoms if you are also taking finasteride. There are two methods in which tadalafil can be given to treat erectile dysfunction (ED). The optimal method of administering tadalafil to you will be decided by your doctor. The exact amount you should take is dependent on the method your doctor has prescribed. The first method involves taking it as needed, often thirty minutes prior to engaging in sexual activity. One study found that tadalafil's impact on libido lasted for 36 hours. Another option for erectile dysfunction treatment is to take tadalafil consistently, at the same time each day. In this manner, you are free to engage in sexual activity whenever you like in between doses.

To treat erectile dysfunction and benign prostatic hyperplasia (BPH), take tadalafil once daily or as prescribed by your doctor. You are free to engage in sexual activity whenever you feel the need in between dosages.

Negative Reactions

You might feel queasy, have a stuffy nose, aches and pains in your muscles and back, nausea, vomiting, or even fainting. Notify your healthcare provider without delay if you experience any of these side effects or if they worsen. When getting up from a seated or sleeping position, take it gently to lessen the likelihood of feeling lightheaded or dizzy. Keep in mind that your doctor has recommended this drug because he or she believes the potential benefits outweigh the risks. Serious side effects are uncommon among anyone taking this medicine.

If you already have cardiac issues,

engaging in sexual activity could exacerbate them. Stop having sex and get medical attention immediately if you have heart issues and develop any of the following significant side effects: extreme dizziness, fainting, pain in the chest, jaw, or left arm, nausea. Very rarely, a person may experience a rapid deterioration in vision, leading to eventual blindness in one or both eyes (NAION). Immediately discontinue tadalafil use and seek medical attention if this major side effect develops. Factors that increase the risk of getting NAION include smoking, being over the age of 50, having heart disease, diabetes, high cholesterol, high blood pressure, specific eye conditions ("crowded disk"), and being over the age of 50.

On extremely rare occasions, you may experience a sharp decline or complete inability to hear, along with tinnitus and vertigo. For immediate medical attention, discontinue use of tadalafil if any of these side effects develop. In the extremely unlikely case if you experience an erection that is painful or lasts four hours or more, you should immediately discontinue use of this medication and seek medical attention to prevent long-term complications. Very severe adverse reactions to this medication are uncommon. Itching, swelling (particularly of the face, tongue, and throat), extreme vertigo, and difficulty breathing are all signs of a severe allergic reaction; nevertheless, you should seek medical attention immediately if you have any of these symptoms. The list of potential adverse effects is not exhaustive. Notify your healthcare provider or pharmacist if you have any side effects that are not mentioned above.

BE CAUTIOUS

Cialis, whose generic form is tadalafil, is an erectile dysfunction (ED) and benign prostatic hyperplasia (BPH) drug. Before you use Cialis, there are a few things you should know, just as with other prescription. Discover all the important information about Cialis safety in this all-inclusive guide. We'll go over everything from how to use the medication to possible interactions, side effects, contraindications, and special populations to consider. Safety Measures for Use:

1.Cialis may only be obtained with a doctor's prescription. Only a healthcare professional should prescribe it to a patient so that they can assess the patient's unique needs and decide if it is safe to use.

2.Clinical Indications: Cialis is indicated for the treatment of erectile dysfunction and benign prostatic hyperplasia symptoms. Do not use this product for recreational purposes or if you do not suffer from erectile dysfunction to improve your sexual performance.

3.How Much Cialis to Take: It is very important to take Cialis exactly as your doctor has suggested. Exceeding the dosage instructions could raise the likelihood of side effects without adding any value.

4.Directions for Administration: Cialis is most often taken orally once day, with or without meals, as advised by a healthcare provider. The precise directions for administering the medicine must be strictly adhered to. Warnings Regarding Dosage: 1.Dosage Guidelines: For males experiencing erectile dysfunction, a standard starting dose of 10 mg of Cialis taken 30 minutes before sexual engagement is recommended. Age, general health, and the existence of other medical issues are some of the individual variables that could affect the dosage. 2.Dosage changes may be required for specific populations due to medical issues like liver or kidney dysfunction. Before giving Cialis, doctors should thoroughly review

their patients' medical histories.
Safety Measures for Interactions:
1. Cialis may increase the risk of side effects from other drugs, especially alpha-blockers and nitrate-containing ones (like nitroglycerin). Hypotension, which can be life-threatening, can result from these interactions. If a patient is using any other drugs, vitamins, or herbal remedies prior to starting Cialis, they should tell their doctor.
2. To avoid an overdose, it is best to avoid grapefruit or grapefruit juice while taking Cialis because they both raise blood tadalafil levels.

Avoiding Adverse Reactions:
1. Typical Cialis side effects include a runny or stuffy nose, flushing, muscle soreness, back pain, headache, and indigestion.

Typically, these adverse effects won't last long and aren't too severe.

2.Although severe side effects of Cialis are uncommon, they include priapism (an erection that lasts longer than four hours), blurred vision, or decreased hearing. It is imperative that patients who encounter any of these symptoms promptly consult a medical professional.

Not to be used:

1.People who have an intolerance to tadalafil or any of Cialis's other components should not take the drug.
2.Patients with pre-existing cardiovascular disorders, such as heart disease, should use Cialis with caution because sexual activity can provide hazards to these individuals.
3.Patients who have recently suffered a heart attack or stroke should not use Cialis because of the increased risk of cardiovascular complications during sexual activity.
Target Audiences:
1.Patients above the age of 65 may need lesser doses of Cialis due to increased sensitivity to the drug's

effects.

2.The use of Cialis in children is not recommended.

3.Cialis is not safe to take while pregnant or nursing because it is not made for female users. Finally, for benign prostatic hyperplasia and erectile dysfunction, Cialis is a popular medicine. Nonetheless, this medicine must be used with extreme caution and only under the guidance of a medical professional. For Cialis to be used safely and effectively, it is essential to follow the dose instructions, be mindful of possible interactions and adverse effects, and know the indications when it is not to be used. The 550-word interaction should always be consulted by patients.

Before you take Cialis (tadalafil), you should think about how it can interact with other drugs, alcohol, and even some foods. These interactions have the ability to impact how well the drug works or heighten the likelihood of unwanted side effects. To ensure the safe and appropriate usage of Cialis, it is vital to understand these interactions.

INTERACTION

Before you take Cialis (tadalafil), you should think about how it can interact with other drugs, alcohol, and even some foods. These interactions have the ability to impact how well the drug works or heighten the likelihood of unwanted side effects. To ensure the safe and appropriate usage of Cialis, it is vital to understand these interactions.

Let's have a look at the different kinds of interactions that can happen when using Cialis:

Interactions between Medications: When it comes to nitrates, which are often recommended for diseases involving the heart and chest pain (angina), Cialis should never be used at the same time. When taken together, nitrates and Cialis pose a serious risk of hypotension, which can result in vertigo, fainting, or even cardiac arrest or stroke.

Alpha-Blockers: Cialis may have an adverse effect when taken with alpha-blockers, which are prescribed to treat hypertension and prostate issues. Taken concurrently, they have the potential to drastically lower blood pressure, which in turn might induce side effects like vertigo, lightheadedness, fainting, or headaches. Healthcare providers may adjust the dosage of alpha-blockers prescribed with Cialis to lessen the risk of low blood pressure.

Concurrent use of Cialis with other antihypertensive drugs may increase the risk of hypotension (low blood pressure) because the blood pressure-lowering effects of Cialis may be amplified. When taken together, these drugs require close observation.

The active ingredient in Cialis,

tadalafil, can reach dangerously high blood levels when using drugs that block the enzyme CYP3A4. This could increase the likelihood of negative effects. Some examples of medications that suppress CYP3A4 enzyme activity are itraconazole, clarithromycin, ketoconazole, and ritonavir. It is possible that lower dosages of Cialis will be required when these drugs are taken together.

On the flip side, Cialis's efficacy may be diminished by CYP3A4 inducers due to lower plasma levels of the drug. St. John's wort, phenytoin, carbamazepine, and rifampin are all substances that induce CYP3A4.

Contacts with Substances:

The chemicals included in grapefruit and grapefruit juice increase the blood concentration of tadalafil by inhibiting the enzyme CYP3A4. Both the effectiveness of Cialis and the likelihood of adverse effects may be amplified in this way. If you are using Cialis, you should not eat grapefruit or drink grapefruit juice.

When it comes to food: Meals Rich in Fat: Eating meals rich in fat can slow down the absorption of Cialis, which means that its effects will not be felt right away. It is best to take Cialis on an empty stomach for the best absorption and effectiveness, while it can be taken with or without food.

Interactions with Herbs: Alterations to Cialis Metabolism:

Some herbal supplements, especially those that may interact with CYP3A4 enzymes, might alter Cialis metabolism. In order to prevent such interactions, patients should tell their doctor about any herbal supplements they are using.

Safety Measures:

Always tell your healthcare provider if you are using any other drugs, vitamins, or herbal preparations before you start taking Cialis. All pharmaceuticals, both legal and illegal, as well as nutritional and herbal supplements, fall under this category.

Healthcare practitioners may need to make adjustments to the dosage of Cialis or suggest other treatments for patients taking multiple drugs in order to limit the potential of interactions.

Finally, the efficacy and safety of Cialis can be impacted by interactions with other drugs, substances, and even specific foods. To reduce the likelihood of side effects and make sure Cialis is used correctly, patients should be proactive in sharing their medical history and current prescriptions with their healthcare professional. Cialis (tadalafil) may interact with other drugs, substances, and even some foods, so it's important for healthcare providers to evaluate each patient's unique situation and make educated decisions about the drug's usage. These interactions have the ability to impact how well the drug works or heighten the likelihood of unwanted side effects. To ensure the safe and appropriate usage of Cialis, it is vital to understand these interactions.

Let's have a look at the different kinds of interactions that can happen when using Cialis:
Interactions Between Medications:
1. When it comes to nitrates, which are often recommended for diseases involving the heart and chest pain (angina), Cialis should

never be used at the same time. When taken together, nitrates and Cialis pose a serious risk of hypotension, which can result in vertigo, fainting, or even cardiac arrest or stroke.

2.Alpha-Blockers: Cialis may have an adverse effect when taken with alpha-blockers, which are prescribed to treat hypertension and prostate issues. Taken concurrently, they have the potential to drastically lower blood pressure, which in turn might induce side effects like vertigo, lightheadedness, fainting, or headaches. Healthcare providers may adjust the dosage of alpha-blockers prescribed with Cialis to lessen the risk of low blood pressure.

3.Concurrent use of Cialis with other antihypertensive drugs may increase the risk of hypotension (low blood pressure) because the blood pressure-lowering effects of Cialis may be amplified. When taken together, these drugs require close observation.

4. The active ingredient in Cialis, tadalafil, can reach dangerously high blood levels when using drugs that block the enzyme CYP3A4. This could increase the likelihood of negative effects. Some examples of medications that suppress CYP3A4 enzyme activity are itraconazole, clarithromycin, ketoconazole, and ritonavir. It is possible that lower dosages of Cialis will be required when these drugs are taken together.

5. On the flip side, Cialis's efficacy may be diminished by CYP3A4 inducers due to lower plasma

levels of the drug. St. John's wort, phenytoin, carbamazepine, and rifampin are all substances that induce CYP3A4.

Contacts with Substances:
1.The chemicals included in grapefruit and grapefruit juice increase the blood concentration of tadalafil by inhibiting the enzyme CYP3A4. Both the effectiveness of Cialis and the likelihood of adverse effects may be amplified in this way. If you are using Cialis, you should not eat grapefruit or drink grapefruit juice.

When it comes to food:
1.Meals Rich in Fat: Eating meals rich in fat can slow down the absorption of Cialis, which means that its effects will not be felt right away. It is best to take Cialis on an

empty stomach for the best absorption and effectiveness, while it can be taken with or without food.
Interactions with Herbs:
1.Alterations to Cialis Metabolism: Some herbal supplements, especially those that may interact with CYP3A4 enzymes, might alter Cialis metabolism. In order to prevent such interactions, patients should tell their doctor about any herbal supplements they are using.
Safety Measures:
1.Always tell your healthcare provider if you are using any other drugs, vitamins, or herbal preparations before you start taking Cialis. All pharmaceuticals, both legal and illegal, as well as nutritional and herbal supplements, fall under this category.

2.Healthcare practitioners may need to make adjustments to the dosage of Cialis or suggest other treatments for patients taking multiple drugs in order to limit the potential of interactions. Finally, the efficacy and safety of Cialis can be impacted by interactions with other drugs, substances, and even specific foods. To reduce the likelihood of side effects and make sure Cialis is used correctly, patients should be proactive in sharing their medical history and current prescriptions with their healthcare professional. In order to make educated judgments about the usage of Cialis in each patient's specific scenario, healthcare providers must first evaluate possible interactions.

LAST THOUGHTS

To sum up, tadalafil, better known as Cialis, is a popular medicine for the treatment of erectile dysfunction (ED) and BPH symptoms. Because it has a longer duration of effect than comparable drugs, it provides substantial benefits to people seeking relief from these problems. Be wary of possible interactions, adverse effects, and precautions when using this medicine, as you would with any other.

We have covered a lot of ground in this talk of Cialis, with an emphasis on the side effects, precautions, and interactions that are part of this medication. It is clear that a thorough approach is required to guarantee the safe and efficient use of Cialis, from comprehending the significance of correct dosage and administration to being cognizant of possible interactions with other drugs, substances, and foods.

The combination between Cialis and nitrate-containing drugs is a major warning sign. These treatments are often prescribed to patients with cardiac issues. Cialis and nitrates, when used together, can cause a potentially fatal decrease in blood pressure, highlighting the need for patients and doctors to be completely transparent about all medications.

A higher risk of side effects and higher blood concentrations of tadalafil could result from interactions with other drugs that impact the enzyme CYP3A4, for example, some antifungal drugs and HIV protease inhibitors. It is important to carefully evaluate prescribing Cialis with medications that stimulate CYP3A4 activity because these treatments may impair the effectiveness of Cialis.

It is important to exercise caution when taking Cialis because of the possibility of adverse effects caused by substance interactions, especially with grapefruit and grapefruit juice. To reduce the likelihood of interactions, patients taking Cialis should be informed to stay away from grapefruit products.

Also, watch out for dietary considerations like eating a lot of fat, because that can slow down the start of Cialis's effects. Even though Cialis isn't dependent on food for absorption, some patients find that taking it without meals helps them get the most out of it.

To make sure that certain populations, such the elderly or

those with liver or kidney problems, may safely and effectively take Cialis, dosage changes could be needed. To address the special needs of these patients, it is vital to closely monitor their progress and create personalized treatment programs.

The best way for people and healthcare providers to manage Cialis is for them to work together. Patients taking Cialis should take the initiative to communicate with their healthcare providers about their current prescription regimen, medical history, and any questions or concerns they may have. Similarly, healthcare providers are vital in determining each patient's unique set of hazards, taking interactions into account, and developing individualized treatment programs.

Patients can get the most out of Cialis and lessen the likelihood of side effects by taking the medication exactly as recommended, paying close attention to how it is administered, and being aware of the possible interactions and side effects. Individuals can confidently add Cialis to their treatment plan, which improves their health and quality of life, by making informed decisions and maintaining open lines of communication. Cialis, whose active ingredient is tadalafil, is used to treat erectile dysfunction (ED) and the symptoms of benign prostatic hyperplasia (BPH). Because it has a longer duration of effect than comparable drugs, it provides substantial benefits to people seeking relief from these problems. Be wary of possible interactions, adverse effects, and precautions when using this medicine, as you would with any other.

We have covered a lot of ground in this talk of Cialis, with an emphasis on the side effects, precautions, and interactions that are part of this medication. It is clear that a thorough approach is required to guarantee the safe and efficient use of Cialis, from comprehending the significance of correct dosage and administration to being cognizant of possible interactions with other drugs, substances, and foods. The combination between Cialis and nitrate-containing drugs is a major warning sign. These treatments are often prescribed to patients with cardiac issues. Cialis and nitrates, when used together, can cause a potentially fatal decrease in blood pressure, highlighting the need for patients and doctors to be completely transparent about all medications. A higher risk of side effects and higher blood concentrations of tadalafil could result from interactions with other drugs that impact the enzyme CYP3A4, for example, some antifungal drugs and HIV protease inhibitors. It is important to carefully evaluate prescribing Cialis with medications that stimulate CYP3A4 activity because these treatments may impair the effectiveness of Cialis. It is important to exercise caution when taking Cialis because of the possibility of adverse effects caused by substance interactions, especially with grapefruit and grapefruit juice. To reduce the likelihood of interactions, patients taking Cialis should be informed to stay away from grapefruit products.

Also, watch out for dietary considerations like eating a lot of fat, because that can slow down the start of Cialis's effects. Even though Cialis isn't dependent on food for absorption, some patients find that taking it without meals helps them get the most out of it. To make sure that certain populations, such the elderly or those with liver or kidney problems, may safely and effectively take Cialis, dosage changes could be needed. To address the special needs of these patients, it is vital to closely monitor their progress and create personalized treatment programs. The best way for people and healthcare providers to manage Cialis is for them to work together. Patients taking Cialis should take the initiative to communicate with their healthcare providers about their current prescription regimen, medical history, and any questions or concerns they may have. Similarly, healthcare providers are vital in determining each patient's unique set of hazards, taking interactions into account, and developing individualized treatment programs. Patients can get the most out of Cialis and lessen the likelihood of side effects by taking the medication exactly as recommended, paying close attention to how it is administered, and being aware of the possible interactions and side effects. By making educated decisions and maintaining open lines of communication, individuals can confidently add Cialis to their treatment plan, enhancing their well-being and quality of life.

THE END

www.ingramcontent.com/pod-product-compliance
Lightning Source LLC
Chambersburg PA
CBHW030058230526
45471CB00003B/1146